Sex Drugs
and
Aphrodisiacs

Notice to Reader

Sex Drugs and Aphrodisiacs

Where to Obtain Them
How to Use Them
and Their Effects

by Adam Gottlieb

20TH CENTURY ALCHEMIST

Sex Drugs & Aphrodisiacs
ISBN: 0-914171-56-9
Copyright © 1973 and 1993 by 20th Century Alchemist
(Originally published by High Times/Level Press)

Cover Design : Bonnie Smetts
Cover Photograph : Harlan Ang
Cover reconstruction : Generic Typography

Published and Distributed by:
And/Or Books.
Post Office Box 522
Berkeley, California 94701

For information about the 20th Century Alchemist, write:
Twentieth Century Alchemist
P. O. Box 3684
Manhattan Beach, CA 90266

Contents

Introduction

DEFINING SEX DRUGS AND APHRODISIACS

The word aphrodisiac often arouses well-deserved cynicism, but even more frequently it inspires bright-eyed fascination and passionate gullibility. Through the centuries, fortunes have been made selling useless powders, ointments, charms, chants, and artifacts to the lovelorn and impotent. In this enlightened age, the desperate are no less easy prey for any profiteer who promises the fulfillment of their hopes and fantasies in a gelatin capsule.

Because so much of sexual interest and arousal is of psychological origin, the customer does not always feel cheated. His passive willingness to believe in the product is often sufficient to effect the desired results. Such is the nature of human faith, which can move mountains and even raise erections.

Still, man is a biochemical creature. His thoughts, emotions and perceptions can be altered to extremes within minutes or even seconds with microscopically small amounts of psychoactive chemicals, such as LSD-25 and DMT. In recent years, the sexual behavior of humans and other animals has been altered in the laboratory by chemical means. Many of the hormones in our bodies are involved in our sexual feelings and activity. This is discussed in some detail

1

later in this book under the entry entitled *Hormones.*

In the medical literature of many ancient civilizations and the present-day practices of primitive peoples, we find numerous herbal materials that have been used to overcome various sexual dysfunctions and to enhance the sex act. Active components have been isolated from many of these plants. Biologists are now learning not only *that* they work, but also *why* they work.

For our purposes in this book, we regard as an aphrodisiac or sex drug any substance which can be used to increase sexual energy and desire, promote and help maintain erection of the penis, delay premature ejaculation, relax inhibition without interfering with performance, serve as a tonic for the health of the sexual organs, overcome sexual lassitude and exhaustion, increase the production of sperm, augment sensual awareness, intensify orgasm, or enhance the enjoyment of sex.

WHAT THIS BOOK IS ABOUT

During the past few years, several companies have offered aphrodisiac materials for sale through advertisements in sexually oriented underground papers. These outrageously priced substances are usually "Guaranteed" to revitalize waning sex drives in both sexes, overcome frigidity and pave the way for multiple orgasm in the female, and conquer impotence and premature ejaculation in the male. Some of these promises are rather overstated in view of the following facts: 1) Impotence, frigidity and premature ejaculation are usually of psychological origin; 2) When physical debility interferes with erection, potency, staying power or enjoyment, it is best overcome by corrected nutrition, adequate rest, reduction of tension, suitable exercise, and refraining from harmful substances, such as alcohol, tobacco, excess coffee, and deleterious drugs. Severe physical defects which interfere with sexual activity are best treated by a medical specialist; 3) Although some of these materials such as ginseng and gotu kola are beneficial to health and may be taken regularly, many others are powerful plant drugs which may be valuable on occasion, but should not be continued to the point of dependency.

We feel that most of these aphrodisiac suppliers are irresponsibly failing their fellow human beings on several grounds: by not clarifying the above-mentioned facts, by drastically overcharging for their products, and by not stating the contents of their products along with appropriate warnings about misuse.

In this book we will tell you what these aphrodisiac substances are, what effects they have, how they work, how to use and not abuse them, and the names of legitimate suppliers from whom they may be purchased at a fraction of the prices charged by the rip-off companies.

We have also included detailed discussions of other sex drugs which are not presently being sold through the aphrodisiac mail order ads. Some of these are illegal in the United States. Others may soon be outlawed.

The various sex drugs and aphrodisiac materials in this book are discussed in alphabetical order. The first sentence of each entry briefly defines the substance: what it is, where it comes from, etc. Some of the entries are fairly lengthy, where there is available information of sufficient scientific, historical or sociological interest to warrant extended discussion. Entries are given on several substances which are presently illegal in the USA (e.g. cannabis, cocaine and opium). This is done because they have attracted considerable interest among the public. Although the author has described various methods of their employment in great detail, this should not be construed as encouragement or endorsement by the author or publisher of their use. The book is written in the belief that humanity has the right to information and knowledge even when these have potential for abuse. It is our hope that the reader will learn from us how to avoid the abuse of the aphrodisiacs and sex drugs which we describe. Furthermore, we are not prescribing any of these substances, legal or otherwise, to our readers. Therefore, we can in no way be held responsible for any mishaps or failures which may occur through the use or misuse of any of these materials or the information which we have supplied.

Encyclopedia
of Sex Drugs
and
Aphrodisiacs

ENCYCLOPEDIA
OF SEX DRUGS
AND APHRODISIACS

ABELMOSK

Also known as musk seeds, abel musk, and moschus grains; the seeds of the bushy herb *Hibiscus moschatus* or *Abelmoschus moschatus* of the mallow family and native to tropical Asia and the East Indies. These musky-scented seeds are used in perfumery, the liquor industry and in flavoring coffee. In India a tincture of the seeds is given orally to counteract hysteria and nervous disorders. The seeds, or a concentrated extract, are also used to overcome hoarseness and as an aphrodisiac. Little is known as to how they manifest their therapeutic effects, but they are regarded as quite reliable.

ABSINTHE

A green-colored liquor flavored with oil of wormwood (*Artemisia absinthium*), anise (*Pimpinella anisum*), marjoram (*Origanum majorana*), elecampane (*Inula helenium*) and other herbs. Absinthe can have an

7

almost instantaneous aphrodisiac effect on both men and women. It also has a strong narcotic effect. When it is taken regularly, it can be damaging to the brain, nervous system, and internal organs. Long-term use can also lead to habituation and be destructive to sexual potency. Insanity can result from its abuse. Used very occasionally and in small amounts, it can be a useful stimulant to the appetites for both food and sex. It is the wormwood oil which is responsible for both the stimulating and harmful properties of this liquor—and the alcohol, of course.

Although wormwood herb grows wild throughout the United States and Europe and is available from legitimate herb vendors everywhere, the liquor and pure oil are illegal in most countries. The herb itself is harmless and is even of medicinal value as a treatment for appetite loss, to dispel worms from the intestines, and to improve mother's milk. The tops of the plant are more potent than the lower portions and are sometimes employed as a cerebral stimulant. The oil contains absinthine, anabsinthin and thujone. In all but small amounts the latter is quite toxic and can cause convulsions and gastro-intestinal disturbances. To summarize: absinthe may make the heart grow fonder, but it can make the rest of the body disintegrate.

AMYL NITRITE

A volatile liquid which acts as a smooth muscle relaxant. It is sold by prescription for controlling heart spasm and to relieve certain types of asthma attack. It is sold in small glass ampules, which must be broken open and inhaled. The usual medical dose is 0.2 ml. More than this causes rapid pounding of the heart and flushed skin. This effect lasts but a few minutes. During this time, it also breaks down inhibitions in much the same manner as nitrous oxide (laughing gas) and relaxes the sphincter muscles. Some people inhale it during sex to produce such relaxations and to enhance feelings of the body. It is also used at the moment of climax to lengthen and intensify orgasm. Amyl nitrite ampules, or poppers as they are often known, are most popular among the gay set. They are frequently used to facilitate the penetration of the anus with the penis or hand. There are usually no unpleasant after-effects from the use of this substance. The odor of amyl nitrite is somewhat reminiscent of rotting apples or pears, which some find distasteful. Amyl nitrite has hypotensive (blood pressure decreasing) effects. Because of this it may be dangerous when used by persons suffering from low blood pressure.

BASIL

This common kitchen herb is the leaves of the plant *Ocimum basilicum* of the mint family. It is very popular in Italy because of its virtues as a seasoning and also because many Italian men claim that eating large quantities of the herb can increase the size of the penis. We have no conclusive evidence that this is so, but if anyone wishes to try it, there can be no harm in the experiment. It may have to be used regularly for a long period of time if results are to be achieved, and, of course, there is no guarantee that it will work. Perhaps it may be effective if the use of the herb is commenced prior to puberty, during which time growth of the genitals occurs. To prove this conclusively, a controlled experiment would have to be conducted upon identical twins. It may be simply that the essential oils in basil act as a mild urethral irritant and cause a more or less perpetual state of mild tumescence in the organ, giving it the appearance of increased size. If it works, it is probably best to use fresh leaves, which can be grown at home or purchased in some Italian produce markets. These can be added abundantly to salads. The dried herb can be sprinkled liberally upon almost any dish, or a strong tea can be made by steeping the herb in boiled water. A liqueur can be made using the same method described under damiana, but substituting basil leaves instead. Good luck—may you add inches to your life.

BETEL NUTS

A piece of areca nut from the Asian palm tree, *Areca catechu*, wrapped in a leaf from the betel vine (*Piper chavica betel*), with a pinch of burnt lime (hydrated calcium oxide), a sprinkle of gambier, obtained from the Malayan woody vine *Acacia catechu*, and a dash of nutmeg, cardamom, turmeric or cloves for flavoring. Betel morsels are sold in the streets and marketplaces of Asia. The morsel is held in the cheek and sucked on for hours like candy. Areca nuts contain a volatile oil called arecoline, which acts as an excitant to the central nervous system. It increases respiration and decreases the work load of the heart. The lime, in combination with saliva, releases the arecoline from the nut. The betel leaf contains several mild stimulants, including cadinene, chavicol and chavibetol. The gambier serves as an astringent and to some extent inhibits the excessive flow of saliva caused by the arecoline.

Areca nuts are gathered by adolescent males and females, who spend their days among the palms alternately harvesting and making love. In 1930, Louis Lewin estimated that there were at least 200,000,000 betel chewers in the world. It is one of the world's most popular drug plants, yet few western people have ever heard of it. In Asian countries it is chewed for its stimulating, spirit-lifting, and aphrodisiacal effects. The latter are due mainly to its general stimulating properties and its ability to increase one's available energy and elevate mood, rather than to any direct influence upon the sexual organs. Excessive arecoline from either immoderation or the use of unripe nuts can cause dizziness, inebriation, convulsions, vomiting, and diarrhea. Regular use eventually stains the mouth deep red. Long-term and immoderate use may eventually weaken sexual potency. Moderate use of the morsel is harmless and may even be beneficial.

BLACK TEA CONCENTRATE

This is made from the dried immature leaves of the Asian shrub *Camellia thea* (formerly known as *Thea sinensis*). Although this tea is consumed throughout the world in moderate amounts (a teaspoon to a cup) for mild stimulation, in China, India and Japan a concentrated extract is often taken for its positive effect upon the sex drive.

Two ounces of tea leaves are boiled in a gallon of water for two hours. The liquid is strained and boiled over a low flame for 24 hours or until it is reduced to a thick syrup. Just a few drops of this syrup may have a strong effect upon the libido. Asian prostitutes sometimes prepare a cup of scented and sweetened water with a few drops of black tea concentrate for customers who are slow to rise to the occasion.

Tea leaves contain 2 to 3% caffeine, which acts as a mild stimulant of the cerebral cortex. They also contain another similar xanthine called theophylline, which dilates the coronary artery carrying blood to the heart.

BUCHU LEAVES

The leaves of any of several *Barosma* species of the rue family growing in Africa. They are usually given as an infusion in water, sherry or brandy and are principally administered in diseases of the genito-urinary organs. They are useful in treating inflammation and catarrh of the bladder and when used for a while afterwards can have a restorative effect on these organs. Buchu is a stimulant and aid to the digestive organs, and has been included in various standard medical preparations, as well as in "secret formulas" of vendors. It has also been credited with the power to delay and, in some cases, reverse the signs of aging, but there is little, if any, substantial evidence to support this notion. It seems at best to be a useful stimulant and beneficial tonic.

BURRA GOKEROO

The oily seeds of the southern Asian plant *Pedalium murex*. It has been used to treat mild infections of the genito-urinary canals, incontinence of urine, and impotence. To prepare it, one part seed is crushed in twenty parts water and three parts pure grain alcohol. This is soaked for 24 hours, strained, bottled, and refrigerated. One teaspoon is taken three times daily. Its effect is to stimulate the spinal ganglia which influence the erectile tissue, in the same manner as strychnine, opium and yohimbine. It appears to be the least toxic of these. Its action is also tonic and antispasmodic.

CACTUS FLOWERS

The commercial name for the stems of the night-blooming Cereus cactus *(Cereus grandiflorus, Mill.)*, which is native to Mexico, southwest USA (American Indians use the root) and Jamaica. It contains a substance with heart-stimulating properties similar in action to digitalis, but unlike that drug in that it is non-cumulative. It has been used to treat several ailments, including prostate disorders, menstrual headaches, weak heart, and sexual exhaustion. To gain increased sexual energy, one may chew ½ gram of the fresh plant material. Or the same amount may be crushed in 2 cc of brandy and allowed to soak for a while before drinking. Since the active drug is alcohol-soluble, this hastens and augments its action.

CALAMUS

The dried root of the semi-aquatic perennial plant of the arum family, *Acorus calamus*. This plant, with its tall sword-like leaves, is found in marshes, stream borders, and ponds of Europe, Asia, and the eastern half of the North American continent. It is also known as sweet flag. It is mentioned in the ancient medical treatises of India as a medicine for many purposes, including the improvement of memory, prolongation of lifespan, and increase of sexual potency. It is similarly used by the Cree Indians of northern Alberta. A piece of root about the thickness of a pencil and two inches long is chewed daily. The essential oil of the root contains asarone, which has 18 times the psychoactive potency of mescaline. A piece at least ten inches long is required to produce any consciousness alterations. Smaller amounts act as a gentle stimulant of the central nervous system.

CANNABIS

Any of the active products of the plant *Cannabis sativa* or *Cannabis indica*. This includes marijuana (the dried flower tops and leaves), hashish (the resinous exudate gathered from the tops or extracted from the plant) and hash oil (any refinement or concentrate derived from the crude extracts, such as brown oil, red oil, or honey oil). These are the forms found in the commercial underground market in the USA. In India and other eastern countries the different cannabis products are ganjah (the resin-covered flower tops), bhang (the leaves from below the tops), charas (the resin gathered from the tops), and hashish or mimea (the resins extracted with fat in water, and solidified). Some of these terms mean different things in different countries. Hashish and bhang sometimes refer to an intoxicating beverage made from cannabis. At present, cannabis products are illegal in many countries, including the United States.

Marijuana is most well-known as a mild psychedelic. It also has a history as a sex drug. In India, aphrodisiac sweetmeats are made from cannabis seeds and leaves combined with musk and honey. Musk, of course, has a fairly sound biochemical basis for its aphrodisiacal potential. It is the sexual attractant produced in the glandular sac beneath the abdominal skin of the male musk deer. Still, there are numerous reports both casual and scientifically documented of marijuana's ability to effect sexual excitement. There are also as many reports that marijuana either had no effect upon sex drive, or even dampened erotic feelings. This is probably due to the fact that different people at different times respond differently to the same drug. Alcohol, for example, makes some people chummy and others belligerent. The aphrodisiacal properties of cannabis are generally credited to its capacity for reducing inhibitions. Any drug which relaxes conscious concerns is likely to have some such effect. Alcohol is one of the most well-known inhibition relaxants. But whether you use cognac or cannabis, this result is anything but guaranteed.

Many people in this civilization are plagued with an abundance of pent-up desires which have been repressed through early training as well as by social and legal condemnations aimed at the adult world. Often, these urges are locked up, but on the very brink of breaking free. In such instances, some mild anti-inhibition catalyst, like marijuana, alcohol, or even visiting a foreign country, will release these pent-up desires and send the individual on a spree of unprecedented libertine activity.

A few years ago Dr. Wesley Hall, president of the American Medical Association (1971–1972), stated that chronic marijuana use can lead to sexual impotence. Naturally, this statement worried many otherwise happy people. Other scientists from all over the world questioned Dr. Hall's remark and wanted to know upon what studies he had based his comment. After some hemming and hawing, Dr. Hall finally admitted that there was no basis for his statement, except that he felt that anything that might discourage the use of pot, whether it be fact or fancy, was justified. Such reasoning from a supposed leader in the medical world boggles the mind. Apparently he could find no substantial fault in marijuana, or he would have surely reported it instead of resorting to a lie. Shortly thereafter a study revealed that sexual activity among pot smokers is 60 to 80 percent higher than among non-users.

Marijuana both stimulates and relaxes the mind and body, and puts the user in a mood for hedonistic pleasures. It does not remove inhibitions to the point of irresponsibility. The notion that it does is largely the result of the prejudicial anti-Mexican and anti-Negro propaganda promulgated by police, politicians, and trashworthy tabloid reporters who began this dubious campaign in the mid-twenties. A person who uses marijuana has complete control over his actions. His inhibitions are merely relaxed to the extent that his mind and body are more free to enjoy the pleasures he chooses.

Occasionally marijuana may set one's mind on an engrossing cerebral journey or draw the user into introspective contemplations. In such a situation, it may divert concentration away from the sex act. It is also possible that if a person is with someone to whom he is not truly attracted, the truth-clarifying nature of the herb will make this fact all too vivid.

On rare occasions the relaxation of inhibitions will be so dramatic that it might seem that critical judgment is lacking. At one time I knew a lady who was ordinarily quite Victorian in her behavior. But whenever she smoked marijuana at a party, she submitted immediately to an urge to fellate every man in the room. So suddenly were her prudish bonds abandoned, that it might easily appear that her common sense had taken flight. This was not the case, however. If any of the males wanted to penetrate her vaginally, she would decline on the grounds that she had a tendency towards pregnancy and did not wish to make any foolish mistakes. Her oral proclivities were no doubt always there, waiting to be freed momentarily from the chains of her pristine up-bringing.

A process for preparing khala-khij, an African aphrodisiac reputed to have liberating and fortifying effects upon men and women, is given in the Stone Kingdom publication, *Drug Manufacturing for Fun and Profit*, available from M.S.A., 417 North Third St., Philadelphia, PA 19123. The procedure involves reinforcing the potency of marijuana with resins extracted from the seeds and stems of cannabis and allowing blue mold to act upon it for several weeks, after which it is dried and smoked.

Methods for vastly increasing the potency of marijuana, hashish and hash oil are described in precise detail in the And/Or Press publication, *Cannabis Alchemy—Making High Potency Hash Oil* by David Hoye, available from Twentieth Century Alchemist, P.O. Box 3684, Manhattan Beach, CA 90266. This book gives practical methods for extracting concentrated hash oil from cannabis products and converting one of the non-active components to active THC while simultaneously transforming the lower rotating delta-8 THC molecule to a higher rotating delta-9 isomer. These two conversions make the hash oil up to six times its original potency, remove the groggy feeling that some cannabis causes, and produce a more aware and spiritual high. These factors are of great importance, of course, when using cannabis as a love sacrament.

CAPSICUM

The dried and powdered fruit of the red pepper *Capsicum frutescens*. This pepper is grown in India, Africa, Japan, the East Indies and tropical America. A most common form of capsicum produced in Mexico is known as cayenne pepper.

Many herbal books recommend capsicum as a healthful nerve and heart stimulant, body purifier and balancer of blood circulation. It has also been used to protect against the common cold. It can be used as a condiment on food. It may cause an intense burning sensation in the mouth, but this does not indicate that it is actually doing injury. It is merely stimulating the nerve endings which are responsible for the sensations of heat. When the "heat"-stimulating oils in capsicum are later passed in the urine, they may cause a mild irritation or tingling sensation of the urethral canal. This may give the illusion of sexual excitement.

Some mail order suppliers of sex stimulants advertise "herbal Spanish fly" or "legal Spanish fly". Real Spanish fly is both dangerous and illegal. Most of these mail order products are simply cayenne pepper in capsules. The supplier frequently charges as much as $20 for a few capsules which the customer could have prepared for himself for less than 50 cents. Cayenne pepper is available at any food market. Gelatine capsules can be purchased at most pharmacies. 30 to 125 mg of capsicum is the usual dose. Some sex stimulant suppliers blend the capsicum with other powdered materials, such as ginseng, kelp, ginger and gotu kola. Some individuals find that straight capsicum, especially when concentrated in a capsule, is upsetting to the stomach. It is best for them to take their capsicum with their food or to blend it with other, more gentle herbs.

CHERRY STONES

The nut-like kernel inside of the pit of the common cherry *(Prunus cerasus)*. They have a slightly bitter taste and a strong odor like that of almond extract. The stones and the tincture from them have been used in herbal preparations for the treatment of coughs, kidney and bladder stones, and spleen disorders. They are also considered to be a cure for impotence in the male. We have found no literature to explain how this cure is effected. The kernels of the cherry, however, like those of its close relative, the apricot, are very rich in vitamins B_{15} and B_{17}. Both of these vitamins are the subject of much controversy recently. There is copious medical literature demonstrating that vitamin B_{15} (pangamic acid) can prevent the degenerative diseases of old age through its ability to bring life-giving oxygen to all of the organs and tissues of the body, and that vitamin B_{17} (laetrile) can control cancer in its early stages and relieve its agonies, even in terminal cases. Still, many state food and drug controls forbid the sale of pangamic acid, and the federal FDA will not permit laetrile to be sold or dispensed by prescription or even tested in hospitals. In the struggle between sincere, devoted medical men and the bureaucrats of the FDA, it has become painfully obvious that the AMA and the FDA are terrified over what these two natural and inexpensive substances would do to medical economics if they were to come into common use. Even now, at the time of this writing, the FDA is trying to enact laws which would forbid the non-prescription sale of all vitamin and mineral supplements.

Both cherry and apricot kernels also contain traces of prussic acid, a deadly poison. The amount of this poison varies with different crops of the fruit. Generally, if the kernel contains dangerous amounts of this chemical, its fruit will be bitter and useless. Trees bearing such fruit are destroyed by the growers. There is no harm, and probably much value in eating a few of these nutritious kernels daily. The toxic component is one that occurs normally in the body's metabolic processes, and is therefore not cumulative.

The Hunza people of the Himalayan region, famous for their long and vigorous lives, make the practice of cracking open the pit of the apricot and consuming its kernel after eating the fruit. They also grind the kernels and bake breads from the meal. Cooking destroys the toxic materials, but leaves most of the nutritional value intact. Cherry kernels must be obtained through the labor of cracking open the stones one at a time. Apricot kernels are available at reasonable prices from some health food stores and from some of the mail order herb companies listed towards the end of this book.

COCAINE

One of several alkaloids found in the leaf of the South American shrub *Erythroxylon coca*. For centuries, the early Incas and later Indians of Peru have chewed the leaves of the coca bush as a stimulant, aphrodisiac and medicine. The drug is a central stimulant and also activates the higher centers of the brain, giving a sense of boundless energy and freedom from fatigue.

In 1859, Albert Niemann isolated cocaine from the coca leaf. This opened up an era of medical and individual experimentation, which flourished until the Pure Food and Drug Law of 1906 and the Harrison Narcotic Act of 1914 made coca and cocaine unavailable legally. It was during this period that Angelo Mariani amassed a fortune selling his popular tonic wine of coca, and that Coca Cola, as it was originally manufactured from "the real thing," became the favorite of the masses. Today illegal cocaine is becoming more popular than ever as· the drug of the elite hedonist.

Of all the illegal drugs, cocaine is the one most often regarded as a sex drug. A snort or two of cocaine can give a person tremendous sexual energy. A man who has taken cocaine may find himself maintaining erection even after several orgasms. The drug also tends to give a man great control over orgasm. This is valuable in chronic cases of premature ejaculation and may be of some use to persons who are trying to develop control in Tantric sex techniques. Even after many orgasms a man who has taken cocaine may still be semi-hard and able to enjoy karezza, the practice

of long, sustained intercourse in which the two part-
ners barely move their bodies but rely upon the more
subtle movements of the pulsations and quiverings of
the sexual organs. The ability of cocaine to permit
lengthy intercourse is so positive that it is advisable
to make use of a lubricant during such episodes. The
female glands which provide lubrication usually dry
out before the experience is completed.

Sometimes, depending upon the individual and his
mood, cocaine may have an opposite effect upon
sexual desire and performance. Occasionally, the
drug will so greatly stimulate the intellectual centers
of the mind that the brain will fairly reel with hyper-
active thought. This can detract from sensual desire
to the extent that all the person may want to do is
think or talk out his thoughts. Cocaine can be a very
"talkative" drug. This can be annoying to a lover if
the subject matter is not of an intimate nature. Most
often, however, the talkativeness manifests itself as
openness and willing communication of personal
feelings. People who are into kinky sex (offbeat,
unusual or even bizarre sexual experimentation
which the taboo-scarred members of our society call
perverted) find cocaine the ideal drug to put them in
the mood for such pleasures.

Cocaine is most often snorted and sometimes injected. To snort it one usually places a small amount
of the drug on the surface of a small mirror and, with
the aid of a single-edge razor blade, arranges two
lines of the material. A line is a pile of cocaine about
½ inch long, $\frac{1}{16}$ inch wide, and $\frac{1}{16}$ inch high. Each of
these is snorted into a nostril through some tubular
device such as a rolled-up dollar bill. Sometimes a

cokespoon is used. Another way to take cocaine is to dissolve it in liquor. About a gram can be dissolved in ⅘ pint of any liquor (Benedictine and brandy is the author's favorite). One tiny cordial glass is sufficient for the desired effect. An even less common way of using cocaine is to smoke it. To do so, one line of the drug can be added to each joint of marijuana or some other suitable material. The cocaine may also be placed on a piece of aluminum foil with a match held under it. As the smoke rises from the cocaine it is inhaled through a piece of tubing. Many coke-and-sex fans claim that smoking cocaine is better for sex than snorting it. It is said to be more effective and reliable in prolonging endurance this way. However, it is not as stoning and its effects do not last as long. Most cocaine comes as the hydrochloride salt. The free-base form, because of its lower melting and evaporation points, is more effective than the hydro-chloride for smoking. When smoking cocaine, one will notice a sensation of numbness in the lungs. This is quite harmless and will soon pass.

Aside from its internal use for stimulating the brain, nervous system and musculature, cocaine is also applied topically as a surface anesthetic to de-sensitize certain areas of the body. It is sometimes mixed with a little water or ointment and applied to the head and shaft of the penis to decrease sensation and prevent premature ejaculation. Cocaine ointment is also used to make anal intercourse easier and in cases of painful vaginal intercourse. Sometimes after one or more orgasms a woman's clitoris will become so sensitive that further stimulation is irritating. A little cocaine on the clitoris will anesthetize this surface irritation and enable the woman to enjoy many more orgasms. Because there is no sensation in the superficial nerves when this is done, the ensuing orgasms are experienced at more profound levels than usual and are more intense and soul-shattering. Because of the current high price of cocaine, it is more economical to use one of the several other less expensive related benzoic esters, such as benzocaine or butacaine sulfate. There are several products in the forms of ointments and aerosol sprays which are designed for these purposes. They usually sell for about $5 per ½ ounce in adult stores and through mail order. A product called *Solarcaine,* which is used for relieving the pain of sunburn and other surface injuries, is available from any pharmacy or supermarket health aid shelf for about $2.59 per 5-ounce can. It can be used for any of the above-mentioned purposes.

In Peru it is coca leaves rather than cocaine that the Indians use daily. The two ounces of leaves that the average Indian chews each day with a piece of slaked lime to release the alkaloids contains about ½ gram of cocaine. Most medical experts who have knowledge of this drug maintain that the leaves are much better than the extracted alkaloid. Homeopathic doctors have often prescribed small doses of coca leaves in cases of physical exhaustion due to sexual excesses.

Prolonged and immoderate use of cocaine, although not addicting in the same sense as heroin or the barbiturates, can lead to psychological dependence. At this point the effects of the drug upon the body and mind are bound to be deleterious. Coca leaves do not have as much potential for dependency and abuse as does the alkaloid itself. Excessive snorting of cocaine can do damage to the nasal membranes and olfactory nerves. More information on cocaine than could possibly be contained in this brief entry can be found in *The Pleasures of Cocaine* by Adam Gottlieb, published by And/Or Press, and available from The Twentieth Century Alchemist.

COTTON ROOT

The root bark of the Asian herb *Gossypium herbaceum*. It contains materials which increase uteral contractions similarly to ergot (but more safely and effectively), ease labor pains, bring on delayed menstruations, and counteract sexual lassitude in both men and women. To prepare the herb for use, boil one pint of water and 2 ounces of cotton root. Let the boiling continue for 3 minutes. Strain, bottle and refrigerate. One wine glass of the liquid is drunk every 3–5 hours. It is wise not to exceed this amount.

CUBEB PEPPERS

The dried unripe berries of the tropical shrub *Piper cubeba*. These berries, and sometimes the volatile oil extracted from them, were at one time used in the treatment of gonorrhea. They have also been used as a stimulant of sexual appetites. The dried berries can be ground in a pepper grinder and extracted into brandy. Cubebs have a stimulating effect upon all of the mucous membranes, and it is doubtless this characteristic which gives them their aphrodisiacal properties. Their taste is pleasantly aromatic although slightly acrid. The resins and the volatile oil are probably the active constituents of the berry. In China an infusion is made from the leaves of this plant and drunk daily for a week or more, and prior to intercourse. This is supposed to stimulate the male organ and strengthen the erection.

DAMIANA

The leaves of a small shrub, *Turnera diffusa* or *T. aphrodisica,* found in Africa, Mexico and southern USA. One or two tablespoons of the dried leaves are steeped (not boiled) in a pint of water. Some persons drink the tea and smoke the leaves at the same time for a mild marijuana-like feeling of relaxation. A cup drunk before retiring promotes relaxation and pleasant dreams, often of an erotic nature. People—especially women—have noted that a cup of the tea, taken an hour or so before having sex, relaxes them and makes them feel more sexy. Damiana taken in moderation over a period of time has a tonic effect upon the sexual organs and the nervous system. This is most effective when it is taken with saw palmetto. Excessive use (numerous cups daily for an extended period) does not have an increased effect, but may be deleterious to the liver. Moderate use is harmless and even beneficial.

In his book, *A Manual of Sex Magic,* Louis T. Culling describes his experiences with damiana. He prepared a drink as follows: two heaping tablespoons of dried damiana leaves are boiled in one cup of water for five minutes, allowed to cool, strained, and drunk each evening for two weeks. Culling, apparently a man of some years, found that during the period of this practice beautiful women paid more than the usual attentions to him. My guess is that the sexually invigorating effects of the herb showed in his manner and made him more attractive to the ladies. Many women find healthy and sexually vigorous older men especially appealing. Culling mentions a liqueur made from damiana leaves and imported from Mexico. He says, however, that this cordial is too mild to have any aphrodisiacal properties. Indeed, this is so, since damiana liqueur contains only a small amount of the herb as a delicate flavoring. I have the recipe for the preparation of an extremely potent damiana cordial. It is especially effective because the alcohol and honey in it greatly aid in the systemic absorption of the active materials.

Soak 1 ounce of dried damiana leaves in 1 pint of vodka for 5 days. Pour off the liquids, strain and filter through a conical coffee filter paper. Soak the remaining alcohol-drenched leaves in ¾ pint of distilled or spring water for another 5 days. Pour off the liquids, strain, and filter as before. Warm the water extracts to about 160°F and dissolve in this ½ to 1 cup of honey. Combine the alcoholic and aqueous extractions. This can be used immediately or aged for a month or so. During aging, a sediment may form as the liqueur clarifies. This sediment is harmless, but if you wish, you may siphon the clear liqueur from it. One or two cordial glasses of the beverage may be taken nightly for the same results as Mr. Culling describes. And it tastes exquisite.

DATURA

Any one of several species of *Datura*, including *Datura stramonium, Datura arborea, Datura metel, Datura meteloides, Datura innoxia, Datura sanguinea,* and *Datura suaveolens.* Some of these daturas are short plants less than a foot high; others are small trees or tree-like shrubs. All of these daturas contain varying percentages of scopolamine, hyoscyamine and atropine. The most well-known species of datura in the United States is *Datura stramonium,* also known as Jimson weed. It can be found growing here on roadsides and in vacant lots. The plant is related to henbane, mandrake, and deadly nightshade, which contain the same alkaloids in slightly different proportions. All of these plants are employed as hallucinogens and hypnotics. Datura is discussed at great length by Carlos Castaneda in *The Teachings of Don Juan.* The hallucinogenic experience with this material is not often a pleasant one. Supposedly, if a person can stay mentally on top of the psychotropic effects, he can enjoy the sensations of flying to distant places. For most people, however, the experience involves profound dizziness, confusion, babbling, headache, and erratic behavior, followed usually by unconsciousness and complete loss of memory as to what transpired.

Datura and other tropane-bearing herbs have a significant history throughout the world. In Asia the seeds of *Datura metel* are crushed in water and used by thieves to stupefy victims. Whores in India have used it to sedate and rob clients. Many of these whores were previously virgins who had been lured into prostitution by the use of the same drug.

In the Middle Ages, henbane, mandrake and datura were included in witches' brews. An ointment was made from the roots of these herbs boiled in fat—often that of a stillborn child. This ointment was rubbed either on the body or on a broom handle, which in turn was employed as a dildo. The drug was absorbed through the mucous membranes of the vagina or anus, and the broom-handling witch was beset with visions and sensations of flight. The image of a witch flying upon a broomstick is at least partly the result of this practice.

In Ancient Greece and Rome, mandrake root and belladonna (deadly nightshade) were put in wine and served at Bacchanalian orgies. Belladonna, which means *beautiful lady,* was used by women aspiring to that description because it dilates the pupils and lends a fashionable appearance to the eyes.

The use of mandrake for fertility dates back at least to Babylonian times. The Old Testament (Genesis 30: 14–16) tells of Rachel, wife of Jacob, receiving mandrakes from Leah to overcome her barrenness. The root has been used for ages by Oriental women for the same purpose. There is no current scientific evidence that mandrake promotes conception. The fruit of the mandrake has been known as Satan's Apple or Devil's Testicles. This berry, however, seems to be the least effective part of the plant. It is even sold in the Mediterranean region as a gourmet's delight.

All of these plants—mandrake, henbane and deadly nightshade—contain the same alkaloids as datura but in slightly varying proportions. Many of these tropane-bearing plants have been employed in various parts of the world to stupefy virgins and young boys, making them easy prey for seduction—or, more correctly, rape. Aside from the ethical matter of removing an individual's free will, this is also a very dangerous practice. A little too much of the drug, and the victim may spend several days in a coma. Fatality is rare in adults, but thoroughly possible.

Sometimes the drug will have a sort of aphrodisiacal effect, possibly by curtailing self-consciousness and inhibitions. Alcohol may do the same. There may be another biochemical basis for the use of these materials to arouse desire. The British herbalist, Gerard, writes that women with child, upon taking the nightshade, "do often long and lust after things most vile and filthie". Pregnant women, because of the increased flow of certain hormones, are often overwhelmed by strong sexual cravings. The drug may accentuate or release some of these urges. Still, it is difficult to guess what, in Gerard's mind, constituted a thing "most vile and filthie".

Until recently, datura was used in the coming-into-manhood rituals of the Indians of the western Amazon. The boy entering manhood was presented by each of the elders with a datura drink called *maikoa*. If the boy could not drink the required amount, a reed or hollowed bone was inserted in his rectum and the remaining *maikoa* was forced into his bowels as an enema. He would then fall into a sleep or trance, in which he was visited by deceased ancestors, who would instruct him on his duties and expected behavior as a man. The amnesiacal effects of the drug were supposed to wipe away much of childhood's memories and ready the young man for his new life.

Not all of the purposes of these tropane herbs have been for stupefaction, hallucination and seduction. They have also been used medicinally to heal ulcers, scars and inflammations. In India they are reported to have been used to treat pneumonia, heart disease, mumps, epilepsy, and even sex perversion (whatever that may be). Scopolamine, one of the chief datura alkaloids, is used today in non-prescription sedatives and anti-tension preparations. In its hydrobromide form, it is used for overcoming motion sickness. As aphrodisiacs, however, these drugs are most definitely not recommended for popular use.

DITA

The seeds of the East Asian and Philippine tree *Alstonia scholaris*. The bark of this tree of the dogbane family has been used in Asian folk medicine for ages. A tea from the bark reduces difficulties of women's menstrual periods. Sometimes the seeds are combined with the bark to prepare such a tonic drink. The bark, however useful, has no aphrodisiacal properties. The seeds contain a strong alkaloid, chlorogenine ($C_{21}H_{20}N_2O_4$), which stimulates and maintains erection in the male and prevents premature ejaculation. A few grams of the seeds are crushed and soaked in a few ounces of water overnight. On the following day, the liquid is strained and drunk. The exact dosage must be determined on the basis of alkaloid potency in the particular batch of seeds and individual requirements and drug tolerance. Start with two or three grams of seeds and increase dosage a little at a time as needed.

The dita tree has white, funnel-shaped flowers. The bark rolls off the tree in layers, and has long been used by Asian scholars as a kind of parchment on which to write. From this usage the tree gets its Latin last name, *scholaris*.

DMSO

Dimethyl sulfoxide, a solvent substance derived from wood pulp as a by-product of the paper industry. It has the peculiar property of being swiftly absorbed through the skin and into the bloodstream. It may also carry into the system other substances with which it is combined. As it is being absorbed, it produces warmth and stimulation of the area treated. It also relieves soreness in muscles and tendons to which it is applied. A dab of DMSO on the penis can often produce a quick erection in cases of impotence. It should not be taken internally. Neither should it be applied frequently to large surfaces of the body, since excessive amounts of DMSO can have damaging effects upon the kidneys. When DMSO is absorbed into the body, it may cause a garlic-like taste in the mouth. Although the medical use of DMSO is currently proscribed, except for veterinarian use, non-medicinal (industrial) grades of the solvent are available from many chemical companies.

EPHEDRA

A leafless desert shrub, various species of which are found in different parts of the world. From China comes a plant drug known as *Ma Huang,* or *Ephedra vulgaris,* as it is known botanically. This plant contains the alkaloids ephedrine and nor-pseudoephedrine, both of which are chemically similar to adrenalin and have some psychoactive properties. *Ma Huang* has been used for centuries in the treatment of bronchial congestion, hay fever and asthma. Today, it is still medically accepted for these purposes throughout the world. Ephedrine is usually produced for pharmaceutical purposes in its sulfate form.

Another species of the same genus is *Ephedra nevadensis,* which grows in the semi-desert areas of central and southwestern USA. It is commonly known as Mormon tea. This name is something of a derogation of the Mormon lifestyle. The herb was at one time believed to be useful in the treatment of syphilis. The insinuation is that because of the polygamous practices of the early Mormons, these people must have constantly fallen victim to this disease. Ephedra has no ability to cure or alleviate syphilis, but there is some indication that it is useful in the treatment of certain mild genito-urinary inflammations.

Another species, *E. pachyclada,* grows in the mountains of northwest India. In the Khyber region and Afghanistan, this herb is boiled in milk and drunk as an aphrodisiac.

FALSE UNICORN ROOT

The bitter-tasting root of the plant *Helonias dioica,* of the lily family. This root is usually prepared as a fluid extract for the treatment of leukorrhea. It is also employed to stop involuntary discharges of semen (spermatorrhea). It acts as a tonic against weakness of the sexual organs.

FLEECEFLOWER ROOT

The tuber-like root of the Chinese plant known in that country as *shoo koo* or *ho shou niao,* and botanically as *Polygonum multiflori.*

In their book *Chinese Folk Medicine,* Wallnofer and Rottauscher state that this plant medicine restores strength to the liver, bones and muscles, increases the production of sperm, and promotes fertility. Dr. Leung Kok Yuen of the North American College of Acupuncture says that fleeceflower root strengthens the liver, blood, nerves, muscles, kidneys, and reproductive system, nourishes the hair, and is a postnatal tonic for females and a treatment for leukorrhea.

The tuber of the fleeceflower, as it comes whole and in dried form from herbalists, is hard like a rock. Some herb dealers can supply it in powdered form. This is much easier to use. Simply boil the powder in water (about a teaspoon per cup) for several minutes and it is ready to drink. If only the whole root is available, it must be boiled for an hour or more until it is soft enough to mash or break into smaller pieces. These pieces and the boiled liquids are then run through a blender until the tuber particles are reduced to a pulp. The liquids are next filtered through cloth or paper. The taste is not bad. The tubers are usually dried in a smoke oven, which imparts a pleasant hickory-like flavor to the material.

Another method is to make an alcohol extract of the tuber with vodka or brandy. To do so, several small tubers are combined with the alcohol in a blender and reduced to splinters. This mixture is put in a jar, allowed to sit and soak for a week, and then filtered. More alcohol can be added to the remaining pulp for a second extraction. After this has soaked for a week, it is filtered, the pulp is discarded, and the liquids are added to those from the first extraction. Sometimes, similar extractions are made of ginseng and gotu kola and combined in equal parts with the fleeceflower extractions.

Whether the decoction is made in alcohol or water, the herb does not bring instant results. It must be taken once or twice daily for several weeks before its effects are noticeable.

FO-TI-TIENG

The fan-shaped leaves of the Asian marsh pennywort (*Hydrocotyle Asiatica minor*). The name *fo-ti-tieng* in Chinese means "elixir of long life". Asians have used this herb for exactly that purpose. There is much evidence of its effectiveness. The most famous case is that of the Chinese herbalist, Li Chung Yun, who according to Chinese government records was born in 1677 and died in 1933 (256 years old). He was living with his 24th wife at the time of his death. One tends to doubt the accuracy of his birth and death records, but it is certain that the man did live an unusually long life and retained most of his vigor nearly to the end. How much of his longevity and vigor was due to *fo-ti-tieng* and how much to other causes is hard to say. He followed very stringent dietary habits, such as vegetarianism and fasting. He raised his own food. But he also used *fo-ti-tieng* in combination with ginseng daily. Jules Lepine, the French biochemist, found in the plant an alkaloid which can have a rejuvenating effect on nerves, brain, and endocrine glands. It has since been found that this substance stimulates a portion of the adrenal glands which detoxifies impurities in the body. Daily use of ½ teaspoon of the powdered herb in a cup of hot water has excellent effects: improved digestion, resistance to disease, calming of nerves, increase of mental and physical energies, and softening of the signs of aging. Larger amounts such as 1–2 tablespoons daily act as a sexual stimulant when sexual vitality is at a low. Continued use has beneficial cumulative effects. There is some argument among botanists as to whether this plant and gotu kola (*Centella Asiatica*) are different species or merely geographical variants. The latter is a slightly larger plant which is found in Ceylon, India, and parts of Africa. Our own experience indicates that, at least for nutritional and medicinal purposes, the two plants may be regarded as identical. Many people feel that the best results are experienced when fresh gotu kola or *fo-ti-tieng* leaves are used. The plant is easy to cultivate. It requires moderate shade and plenty of water (it is a marsh plant). Just a few plants will send out runners and spread like strawberries, if conditions are right. The leaves have a tangy flavor. Two or more can be chewed daily for maintaining vigor and as a psychic energizer. More may be taken for immediate stimulation of the libido. A source of live plants is given at the end of this book.

FUGU

A preparation, popular in Japan, made from the testes of a species of poisonous puffer fish found in many oceans. A tablespoonful of the milky testicular fluid is mixed with a cup of hot *sake* and drunk. It is apparently a very potent sex stimulant, but sometimes it may act as a powerful and deadly nerve poison. If this is the effect which it has on a person, he will feel numbness in his extremities soon after drinking the cocktail. He may collapse shortly thereafter, suffer breathing difficulty, and eventually heart failure. This aphrodisiac is popular only in Japan, where it claims about 300 lives annually. There is no known antidote for the poison. Perhaps, if the aphrodisiacal component is other than the neurotoxin, it can be extracted or synthesized. If the two effects are caused by the same component, it may be that concentrations vary. In this case, isolation of the active substance would give better control of the dosage.

GARLIC

The bulbs of the common kitchen herb *Allium sativum*. It is regarded as one of the healthiest foods on earth. It acts favorably on the metabolic processes and frees the bowels and blood vessels of deposits. One who uses garlic regularly usually feels very fit. The Ammites of China are among the most lusty people in the world. They credit their good health and powerful sexual vigor to the large amounts of garlic that they use. The same is true of some of the Russians who inhabit the Caucasus region and usually live to be robust centenarians. In India, men often rub ointment made from garlic and fat on the penis and lower back to promote and maintain a powerful erection. It should be pointed out that the fragrance of garlic does not usually serve as an erotic stimulant to the partner of one who has consumed it in quantities or rubbed it on his body.

GINSENG

The root of the Asian plant *Panax schinseng*. It is used by Oriental men to prolong life, retain virility, increase and regulate the flow of hormones, strengthen heart, nerves and glands, reduce susceptibility to disease and toxins, and improve circulation and sexual potency. The ancient Vedic medical books of India claim that ginseng "bestows on men both young and old the power of a bull". Ginseng contains panaquilon (stimulant of internal secretions), panaxin (central organ, heart and blood vessel stimulant), panacene (stimulant of medulla centers and relaxant of nervous system), and panaxic acid (promotes metabolism and relaxes heart and artery movements). Other constituents are amylase and phenolase (enzymes), vitamins B_1 and B_2, schingenin, and saponins. A piece of ginseng about the thickness of a pencil by one inch long may be moistened in the mouth and chewed daily, or the equivalent amount of shavings or slender root tails may be chewed or boiled as a tea. The pulp from this may be boiled over and over again. Later, the remaining pulp may be chewed and swallowed. Because saliva helps to release and activate the constituents, it is best to sip the tea slowly and allow each sip to linger in the mouth for a minute before swallowing. Some herbalists believe that ginseng is more effective when taken with gotu kola (*fo-ti-tieng*). The best quality ginseng available commercially is from Korea, because it is government-controlled. Much ginseng imported from Hong Kong is merely American ginseng (*Panax quinquefolium*) disguised to look like the Korean type. American ginseng has many values too, but lacks the potency of the Korean variety. It is not bad if you are paying for American rather than Korean.

GUARANA

The seeds of the South American woody liana *Paullinia cupana*. They are gathered in October, ground, sometimes mixed with cassava flour, made into a paste with water, and dried in the sun. Often the paste is shaped into sticks and dried over fire. When an energizing drink is needed, half a teaspoon or so of guarana powder is grated from the stick and added to a cup of hot or cold water. Guarana is frequently sold through mail order ads as a stimulating aphrodisiac. The stimulation is due to the presence of twice as much caffeine as is in coffee. Guarana is also used as a tonic and nervine against headache and neuralgia due to menstrual disorders.

HENNA

The leaves of the Old World tropical shrub *Lawsonia inermis*, of the loosestrife family. Today, as through the ages, henna leaves are used to dye the hair red and sometimes to tint the fingernails. In India, powdered henna is rubbed several times daily on the skull, fingertips, and soles of the feet for several weeks as a cure for impotence and premature ejaculation. It is true that these parts of the body are excellent points of absorption, but there is no present knowledge as to what substances in the plant are responsible for the alleged efficacy of this cure.

HORMONES

The action of hormones is to stimulate other actions in the body. Some hormones stimulate the production of other hormones. The pituitary serves as a master gland, dispensing precise amounts of various hormones into the bloodstream, which have a direct effect upon behavior and also govern the flow of other hormones. Some of these other hormones have a reciprocal influence on the pituitary secretions. Much of the maleness or femaleness of the individual is determined by the pituitary. The so-called sex hormones are mostly produced in the sexual organs and the adrenal cortex. In the male these are generically known as androgens and include such well-known substances as testosterone and androsterone. The female hormones include estrogens and progestins. The body produces hormones of the opposite sex, but usually in lesser proportions than those of its own sex. Androgens produced at puberty stimulate development of secondary sexual characteristics, develop and maintain the testes and the production of sperm, produce a positive nitrogen balance which assists growth and improves muscle tone, and may increase the size of underdeveloped genitals.

Androgen preparations such as testosterone propionate (injectible) or methyltestosterone (oral) have been given in cases of deficiency to bring on secondary sexual characteristics and to delay male climacteric. Undesirable side effects may include acne, baldness, sodium and water retention, hypercalcemia, and, in the case of methyltestosterone, liver damage. Androgens are sometimes given to women as a treatment for breast engorgement and cancer. Side effects may include development of male characteristics, such as facial hair, sinewy muscles, husky voice, and decrease of breast size, as well as some personality and behavioral changes. Transsexuals (persons who have had their sexuality altered surgically) are given a lengthy series of hormones to complete the conversion. Testosterone is also used in the treatment of impotence. It should be taken only under the guidance of a qualified endocrinologist. One of the dangers in the regular use of testosterone and related hormones is that the body may become dependent upon the medicine and slow down its own production of these hormones.

Other hormonal substances may have considerable influence upon sexual behavior. Human chorionic gonadotropin, which is produced during pregnancy, can cause increase of sexual desire in the female. For this reason, many women become very horny when they are with child. Synthetic androgens such as Dianabol (methandrostenolone) and other anabolic agents which are given for weight gain in undernourished patients frequently cause an increase in libido as a side effect. These drugs have been used to excess by weight lifters and body builders who sought remarkable gains in muscularity. This has often led to a serious disruption of the balance of the entire endocrine system.

Generally, the best way to keep the body's hormones balanced and flowing is to maintain good mental and emotional health and to treat the physical body right through proper rest, regular exercise, adequate diet, and minimizing the use of harmful substances, such as coffee, alcohol, tobacco, amphetamines, and barbiturates. Occasionally, when needed, herbs which contain hormones may be taken. These include sarsaparilla, licorice, hops, and pollen.

IBOGA

The roots (especially the root bark) of the equatorial African forest shrub, *Tabernanthe iboga*. The powdered bark is consumed by the natives of Gabon in their Bwiti ritual, in which they communicate with the ghosts of departed ancestors. It is also chewed before the lion hunt. The drug enables the hunter to remain awake while standing motionless for as much as 48 hours. In this position he patiently waits for the lion to cross his path.

It is also used as an aphrodisiac and cure for impotence. Its efficacy as a sex drug is borne out by my personal experience and that of others. There are many instances in which persons, after consuming a gram or so of the bark, engaged in nonstop sexual activity for periods ranging from 6 to 17 hours.

The bark contains about 6% mixed indole alkaloids. The main component is ibogaine, a stimulant, hallucinogen, and cholinesterase inhibitor. Despite the fact that ibogaine is virtually unknown in the United States and has never been a problem drug, it is illegal in this country.

Sometimes, the African will take other plant drugs along with iboga. One of these is *Alchornea floribunda*, known in Liberia, Nigeria and Uganda as *niando*. The root bark of this shrub of the spurge family is macerated in palm or banana wine and drunk for its stimulating influence on the libido. The effect of *niando* is at first very stimulating. But as the drug wears off, a depression sets in, and sometimes death results. Little study has been done on this herb, but there are indications that its active component is yohimbine. If so, this would explain its severe side effects. Yohimbine is potentiated by alcohol to such a degree that the combination may have fatal results.

KAVA KAVA

The root pulp and lower stems of the perennial shrub *Piper methysticum* from the Hawaiian and South Pacific Islands. The islanders prepare from it a pleasant and harmless narcotic beverage. The drug depresses spinal rather than cerebral activity and therefore produces a euphoric state and relaxation without impairing mental alertness. Its action is due to the presence of six resinous alpha pyrones: kawain, dihydrokawain, methysticin, dihydromethysticin, yangonin, and dihydroyangonin. None of these are water-soluble. They must either be emulsified into water or coconut milk by prechewing the root, as is done in the islands, or by adding a little salad oil and lecithin and mixing it up in a blender. To do this, mix one ounce of powdered kava-kava, ten ounces of water, two tablespoons of coconut or olive oil, and one tablespoon of lecithin granules (available at health food stores) in a blender until it attains a milky appearance. This amount serves two to four persons.

Some people claim that after drinking kava-kava they experience delightfully tingling sensations in the genitals which enhance sexual pleasure. This tingling response is not always the case, however. A resinous tar can be extracted from the root with hot alcohol and evaporation of the solvent in a heat bath or double boiler. A piece of this tar about the size of a pea can be placed on the tongue, and, as it begins to dissolve, it will cause a tingling and numbing sensation in the mouth, much like cocaine. It has a strong but not unpleasant taste and a cinnamon-like odor. If this bead of tar is kept on the tongue while it is being used to stimulate a woman's clitoris, it will produce a mild numbing of the superficial nerves of that organ, which can give rise to profound and delicious feelings for the woman. Frequently, after one or more orgasms—especially if they are clitorally stimulated—the nerves near the surface of the clitoris will become distractingly oversensitive, to the point of seeming sore. If a woman can somehow get past this hypersensitivity, she will at this point of arousal be able to experience some of the most wildly ecstatic and deeply moving orgasms of her life. By lightly desensitizing the surface nerves, sensation is transferred to the deeper, underlying nerves. She may then experience voluptuous and soul-probing sexual feelings which are not otherwise possible. Cocaine is similarly used on the clitoris, but its anesthetizing effect is more thorough and is often experienced as a cold numbness. Because of the complex chemistry of kava-kava, its effect is more of a warm, tingling numbness which produces enjoyable sensations even without the benefit of oral stimulation.

KELP

An edible seaweed *(Macrocystis pyrifera)* found in several places, including the coastal waters of the Pacific. Because it grows in the sea it contains a perfect balance of organic minerals, and can be used as a salt substitute. These minerals are essential to glandular health. It has in it ten times the iodine of iodized salt. Iodine is necessary for the proper function of the thyroid gland. This gland produces the hormone thyroxin, which is needed to convert carbohydrates into energy. Lack of iodine can result in chronic mental and physical fatigue, irregular and excessive menstruation, and lowered sex drive. One teaspoon of kelp daily will correct most thyroid disorders that were due to iodine deficiency. It may even overcome some forms of obesity.

Other substances which work hand in hand with iodine to promote thyroid health are protein and vitamins C, E, and the B complex group. A tasty and healthful table seasoning, which I call Super-Vita-Shake, can be made by combining five parts powdered kelp with four parts ascorbic acid powder (vitamin C), three parts paprika, two parts onion powder, and one part garlic powder. Shake these well together. Sea kelp is available in bulk form from most health food stores for about $1 per pound. Many of these stores also carry powdered vitamin C in jars at about $10 per pound. Vitamin and mineral supplements are not efficiently assimilated when taken as pills or capsules. The natural way to assimilate any nutrient is along with the food you eat. Super-Vita-Shake is a delicious and nutritious salt and pepper substitute and much more. The kelp gives it a lightly salty taste without supplying the excessive concentrated sodium of common table salt and sea salt. Kelp has a distinctive flavor of its own which adds to the flavor of most dishes. The vitamin C lends a pleasant acidy tang like that of a dash of lemon juice. The paprika supplies rutins and other so-called C complex factors, which are necessary for the body to get the proper use out of vitamin C. The onion and garlic furnish some minerals and B vitamins. Each also has its own flavor, which in combination balances the taste and tang of this condiment. In the future, as people become more aware rather than emotional about nutrition, we will be more inclined towards taking our extra vitamins in this manner. Other powdered water-soluble vitamins, minerals and spices may be combined with Super-Vita-Shake to suit individual and family requirements.

Another excellent way to take kelp is to prepare a tonic drink by mixing one teaspoon of kelp, ⅓ teaspoon (1000 mg) vitamin C powder, one teaspoon of wheat germ oil, and one tablespoon of brewer's yeast or any nutritional yeast in an eight-ounce glass of tomato juice. Shake well or mix in a blender. This combination is somewhat richer in B complex vitamins than the Super-Vita-Shake. The wheat germ oil provides vitamin E, which the shake does not contain.

Because kelp is a concentrated source of nutritional factors rather than a drug, its effects are cumulative, not immediate. After a week or so of use, a person may notice a substantial increase in sexual drive as well as general energy. There is no advantage in trying to cram large quantities of this food in order to hasten its benefits. This could even be dangerous because the body is not prepared to handle so much iodine at one time.

Another seaweed which contains much the same values as kelp is dulse *(Halymenia edulis* and *H. palmata).* It is a perfectly balanced source of minerals and is found along the coast of Britain. Like kelp it can be purchased at most health food or herb shops.

KOLA NUTS

The seed of the African tree of the Chocolate tree family, *Cola nitida.* The seed contains about the same percentage of caffeine as coffee (2%) plus the essential oil. This oil gives the seed its familiar cola flavor and also has stimulating and metabolism-regulating properties. The natives of North Ashanti and Sierra Leone chew the nuts to combat fatigue and to stimulate sexual energies. One can moisten a nut in the mouth and suck on the juices or make a beverage by boiling the broken seeds in water for ten minutes. One heaping tablespoon of the broken seeds to a cup of water is an average dose. Some herb dealers sell the kola nuts in powdered form. One teaspoon or more of the powder can be made into a slurry with a little hot water and then further dissolved in more hot water to make one cup. Honey may be added to sweeten and bring out the flavor. Some people like to add cream. Used in moderation, this beverage can be pleasantly stimulating. It should be remembered, however, that excessive use of caffeine over long periods can be debilitating to the sexual function.

L-DOPA

The levo-rotary (left-handed) isomer of dihydroxy-phenylalanine, also known as levodopa or Laradopa (registered trademark of Roche Laboratories). It is primarily used in the treatment of Parkinson's disease. It has been frequently noted that its use causes increased sexual desire in some individuals. It may also have some very undesirable side effects in some cases, such as nausea, anxiety, depression, confusion, lethargy, blurred vision, hot flashes, and hair loss. It should not be taken by persons who are currently receiving MAO inhibitor drugs, and should be used with caution by pregnant or lactating mothers, persons with an active peptic ulcer, or those who are taking antihypertensive drugs. L-dopa should be taken only under the guidance of a qualified physician. It can be purchased only through prescription.

In recent years, the explanation of L-dopa's sex-arousing properties has come to light. Stress, aging, and other factors can cause increase of the neurohormone serotonin in the hypothalamic region of the brain. This, in turn, has several undesirable effects upon the mind and body. It can increase blood pressure, cause nervous depression and exhaustion, and diminish sexual desire. There is now growing evidence that rises in brain serotonin levels trigger the release of self-destruct hormones, which are partly responsible for the aging process. L-dopa is converted to dopamine in the body. Dopamine is a normal substance in the body and brain. When dopamine levels are high, serotonin levels are low, and vice versa.

Dopamine does not easily pass through the membranous barrier between the bloodstream and the brain. But L-dopa does, and in the brain is converted to dopamine. Under ideal conditions, people should retain healthy sexual appetites late into life, but high serotonin levels lessen the sexual response.

LICORICE ROOT

The sweet-tasting root of the European leguminous plant *Glycyrrhiza glabra*. This well-known substance has a long history as a source of strength and sexual vigor. The Egyptians in the days of the pharaohs made from it a beverage called *mai sus*, which served not only as a refreshment but also as a revitalizing draught for the tired mind and body. The Chinese chewed the root for increased strength and endurance. The Hindus combined a brew made from it with milk and honey and drank it to improve their sexual vigor. To prepare this drink, chop ½ pound of the dried root into small pieces and boil them for five minutes in 3 pints of water. Strain the liquids and boil them down to one quart. This thick, mucilaginous tea is then combined with milk and honey. If the fresh root is available, it is said to be even more effective than the dried root. This beverage is also useful as a soothing agent for gastric ulcers and is helpful in removing flatulence. How licorice root increases sexual energy is not entirely certain at this time, but in 1950 it was found that this root contains a fair amount of the female sex hormone estrogen.

LUPULINE

The yellow or orange powdery gland material from
the strobiles of the hops plant *(Humulus lupulus)*.
This material is separated from the strobiles by shak-
ing the dried flower cones in a closed container. The
lupuline will tend to settle to the bottom. It is used
medicinally to calm the nerves and to encourage
sleep. It also serves as a remedy against premature
ejaculation due to excess sexual excitement. It has a
bitterish taste that some may regard as interesting
but others will probably not appreciate. One or two
teaspoons of the powder can be stirred into a cup of
hot water. A little honey can be added if necessary.
Hops contains minute amounts of the hormone
estrogen. Hops tea can be taken by women to stimulate weak or waning sex glands.

MATICO

The leaves of the South American plant of the pepper
family *Piper angustifolium*. For centuries these aromatic and slightly astringent leaves have been used
by Peruvian Indians as a sex stimulant and general
energizer. They have also been used as a urinary
antiseptic in the treatment of cystitis, gonorrhea, and
catarrh of the bladder. However effective this herb
may be, we cannot recommend the self-treatment of
these disorders. To prepare matico tea as it is used in
Peru, add one tablespoon of the dried leaves to each
cup of boiling water. Allow these to boil for one
minute. Remove them from the flame. Let the pot

stand for thirty minutes. Strain the liquids and permit them to cool. Serve this infusion chilled.

METHAQUALONE

A sedative and hypnotic agent, chemically unrelated to other sedative hypnotics. This drug, whose chemical name is 2-methyl-3-o-tolyl-4(3H)-quinazolinone, is sold by prescription under such names as Quaalude, Sopor, Parest and Mandrax. The usual dose is 150–300 mg for sleep, or 75–150 mg for daytime sedation. Many people who have used methaqualone have noted that it makes them feel very sexy, and enhances sensuality and the sexual experience. Many women who ordinarily lack interest and energy for sex become most desirous of erotic pleasures after taking the drug. It also tends to relax inhibitions to a great extent. While the exact mode of sedative action in methaqualone is not fully understood, it appears to act upon a different central nervous system site than the barbiturates and other hypnotic drugs. Tolerance to methaqualone develops quite rapidly and can lead to addiction. The mind and body become extremely loose under the influence of the drug. Driving is not recommended. Some people experience hangover accompanied by blurred thinking after using methaqualone. These side effects are more likely to occur if one has been taking the drug for a period of time. Death has occurred following overdosage, but most fatalities have followed overdoses accompanied by alcohol.

MUIRA PUAMA

The wood shavings of the South American tree *Lyriosma ovata*. It contains a resin which has strong stimulating effects upon the central nervous system and libido. The natives of the Amazon and Orinoco basins chew the bark or boil it to make a potent beverage. The standard preparation is to boil 2 to 4 tablespoons of the shaved wood for 15 minutes in 1 pint of water. One cup of the strained liquid is drunk 1 to 2 hours before coitus. It should be pointed out, however, that the resin is not water-soluble and that this method neither succeeds in extracting all of the resins, nor are they readily assimilated into the system in this water-suspended form. It is better to extract 4 tablespoons of the shavings into ½ pint of boiling vodka for 15 minutes, strain while hot and drink 1 or 2 cordial glasses ½ to 1 hour before coitus. Or the resin can be extracted into hot isopropanol or any alcohol, strained, and the solvent evaporated in a double boiler or heat bath. The remaining resin is then gathered and refrigerated. One pellet of this material about the size of a pea can be placed in the mouth 1 to 1½ hours before coitus and allowed to dissolve in the saliva before it is swallowed.

NUTMEG

The seed of the tropical evergreen *Myristica fragrans*. It is a common spice found in any grocery or supermarket. Yemenite men in Arabia chew considerable amounts of nutmeg daily because of its alleged ability to increase virility. A few pinches of nutmeg each day can do no harm, but large amounts (5 grams or more) may cause some very undesirable side effects such as: nausea, intoxication, bloodshot eyes, constipation, and difficulty in·urination, followed by a day of sluggishness. Daily use of such doses can be harmful to the liver. Nutmeg contains several psychotropic substances: myristicin, elemicin and safrole. It is sometimes used for its consciousness-altering effects, but usually only when nothing else is available—in prisons, for example.

OPIUM

The dried latex-like exudate of the opium poppy (*Papaver somniferum*). Crude, commercial opium usually takes the form of a black tar with a characteristic odor and rather bitter taste. The drug is often associated with erotic fantasy. Indeed, it can bring to the user wildly voluptuous thoughts, sensations, visions, and dreams. It has, in moderate doses, a stimulating effect upon the spinal ganglia associated with erection, similar to that of strychnine, yohimbine and burra gokeroo. It has a relaxing and sedative effect upon the body and mind in general, but is stimulating to erotic feelings on both the mental and physical levels. It also has a mild anesthetizing effect upon the surface nerves of the glans penis. This is not enough to interfere with the sensations of sex. In fact, it can increase these sensations by delaying ejaculation and allowing the development, during sex, of the deeper stimulation and gratification of the underlying nerves reaching to the very soul of one's erotic being.

Orgasm in both the male and female is more deeply and intensely satisfying if the erotic sensations are allowed to build up slowly and steadily during the sex act. If this is not done, the sensations of orgasm are likely to be more superficial. On the other hand, if there is a steady and gradual crescendo towards orgasm, the entire solar plexus becomes suffused with blood and charged with neural energy. At least on the physical level, the whole sexual experience becomes deeper and more meaningful, and orgasm, when reached, is overwhelming and totally fulfilling. This ultimate orgasm is best arrived at through patient practice, honesty to one's sexual feelings, exercise of some control or channeling of one's emotional energies, the development of genuine feelings towards one's partner, and mental and physical disciplines in delaying premature discharge. Exercises described in *Sexercises* by Edward O'Reilly are of great value in this regard. For more advanced discipline, the techniques of hatha and tantric yoga are most useful.

Many persons find that certain drugs, such as opium, help to bring about the gradual buildup and total orgasm. If one has had no previous experience with profound orgasm, it may be of some value to utilize a drug of this sort to acquaint oneself with the possibilities. Eventually, however, a person should learn through practice to achieve the same results without dependence upon any such substance.

Furthermore, it should be pointed out that although the occasional use of opium in modest amounts may have pleasant and erotic results, immoderate and excessive use can weaken one's sexual powers. Overuse can also weaken the body in general, reduce resistance to disease, and develop into addiction. Aside from all these natural laws concerning opium, there are also the man-made ones which are equally treacherous. The social and legal prejudices against opium are far more magnified than those against marijuana.

There are several ways to use opium. The most well-known method is to smoke it. If one does not do this correctly, most of the material will be wasted and little if any effect will be experienced. Sometimes a marijuana smoker will add tiny fragments of opium to his grass and smoke this mixture in a pipe or joint. This is a great mistake. The heat of the burning marijuana is too intense. Most of the opium will be destroyed before it reaches the lungs.

Actually, one does not smoke opium; one vaporizes it. One of the best ways to do this is to roll a little piece of opium between the thumb and forefinger into a ball about ⅛ inch in diameter. This is placed in the brass bowl of a long-stemmed pipe (available from head shops). The pipe is tilted at an angle so that the molten opium tar is not drawn into the stem. The flame of a match, candle or alcohol lamp is held beneath the bowl so that it licks just slightly over the top of the bowl. As the bowl heats the tar will melt, swell and bubble. A white vapor will rise from this. At the instant that this vapor appears, one begins inhaling deeply to the bottom of the lungs. The vapor is held for awhile and then slowly exhaled.

The residue left in an opium pipe is known as the dross. Because the dross is so rich in alkaloids, smoking it can give some extra kicks, but habitual use can lead one to an early grave.

Opium may also be ingested. The effects of ingestion are longer in duration but slower to come on (30–60 minutes). A piece of opium about the size of a pea (¼ to ½ gram) can be placed under the tongue and allowed to dissolve slowly while the juices are swallowed. Or the same amount can be dissolved in ½ cup of hot water (opium tea) and sipped slowly. Many people become nauseous shortly after the ingestion of opium. If the drug is taken gradually during a period of 45 to 60 minutes, there is less shock to the system and the nausea can usually be avoided.

Another less common method of use is to take opium rectally as a suppository. This may seem bizarre or even disgusting to many persons within our culture because of social taboos and prejudices regarding the anus and feces. Still, it is a most valid method for taking certain drugs. Drugs taken in this manner are swiftly, effectively and economically absorbed into the system. The initial effects are felt sooner (10 to 20 minutes) this way than when the drug is ingested. There are no digestive acids in the colon to destroy the drug. There is far less likelihood of suffering systemic shock and nausea than when it is ingested. Furthermore, opium seems to manifest its aphrodisiacal properties more efficiently when used in this manner. The proximity of the absorption point in the colon to the prostate gland (in the male), genitalia, and spinal ganglia connected to these directs much more of the drug's effects to these regions. Males have frequently reported that when using an opium suppository they maintain a strong erection for longer than usual periods and find it natural and easy to engage in prolonged intercourse without necessarily arriving at climax.

One acquaintance described the experience: "I felt like a human dynamo. Fucking for over two hours with complete control over my orgasm. I could feel the sex energy building up in my gut and spreading through my whole body. I could have gone on all night; maybe forever, it felt. She must have had twenty orgasms. We were both delirious with love or lust or whatever it was. When I finally decided to come it was like an explosion of light."

When using an opium suppository the bowel should be empty. If it is not, much of the drug will be taken up by the feces and later voided. Some people find it helpful to cleanse the bowel with a small enema before inserting the opium. Next one applies a small amount of Noxema or K-Y Jelly to the anus and into the anal canal. Mineral oil and vaseline are not practical because they can hinder the absorption of the drug into the system. A little lubricant is also applied to the sides of the index or middle finger, but not to the tip. A pea-size pellet of opium is placed on the fingertip. With another finger the anal entrance is gently massaged so that it relaxes and opens rather than tightens and closes. The finger bearing the opium pellet is then carefully inserted and the pellet is pushed all the way to the end of the rectal canal. Sometimes, especially if the opium is fresh, it will melt from the warmth of the rectum before it can be pushed all the way inside. This can be prevented by blending the pellet with some flour or talc. Also, the pellet can be kept in the refrigerator until needed.

Women find that the rectal use of opium stimulates fantasy and sexual desire while relaxing the sphincter muscles of both the anus and vagina. For many centuries in the Orient, opium paste has been applied to the rectal canal to relax the surrounding muscles and make anal intercourse easier. It has similarly been used in the vaginal canal of women for whom normal intercourse was painful.

For these purposes, an anesthetic lubricant can be made by lightly melting one part opium and combining it with eight parts K-Y Jelly or Noxema. A fingerful of this mixture is applied to the anal or vaginal canal ten minutes before intercourse. Immediately prior to penetration, more can be applied to both the male and female organs.

Opium can also be injected. This is risky because of the impurities so often found in the crude drug. Because of the personal prejudice of the author against needles, he has scant knowledge and no experience with this method of use. Therefore, it will not be discussed in this book.

The potency of different batches of opium can vary widely depending upon freshness, regional source, method of processing, presence of adulterants, etc. A person experimenting with this or any drug should cautiously determine the correct amount to use by starting with very small doses and gradually increasing.

PEMOLINE

A synthetically prepared hydantoin group chemical. Its proper chemical name is 2-imino-5-phenyl-4-oxazolidinone. It acts as a mental stimulant with very little central nervous system stimulation. Pemoline was used during World War II by American and British flyers to maintain alertness on long bombing missions. At that time the Nazis were using amphetamines, which they had developed for similar purposes. Pemoline is far safer than the amphetamines. It does not have the dangerous and unpleasant side effects of the latter; i.e., cardiac stress, drying of mucous membranes, tension in neck and facial muscles, rapid development of tolerance, and addictive potential.

The usual dose (20–50 mg orally) gives psychic stimulation for 6–12 hours, often with a surprising degree of bodily relaxation. Taken too soon before retiring, it may cause insomnia. It can promote in a tired mind the higher level of mental concentration necessary for prolonged focus upon and full enjoyment of the sex act. It is used in combination with yohimbine hydrochloride, methyltestosterone and strychnine sulfate in a prescription medicine for the temporary treatment of impotence, known as Potensan Forte, produced by Medo Chemicals, Archway, North London, England. Another form of pemoline, called magnesium pemoline, produced in the USA by Abbott Laboratories, has been used for improving memory and in the treatment of senility. It is sold through prescription under the trade name Cylert.

POLLEN

Grains of clustered microspores from the male sex organs of flowering plants, which serve to fertilize the female ovum to produce seeds. Pollens from numerous species of plants are an excellent and nutritional food. Honey has long been recognized as a food rich in many more components than the sugars which comprise the greatest percentage of this substance. This is because of the presence of pollen. Highly refined and filtered honeys have very little of this wonder food remaining in them, and in cooked honey many of the valuable components are destroyed. Pollen is rich in proteins, minerals, vitamin C, and B complex vitamins. It also contains substances which promote the production of sex hormones. Pollen is sweet and pleasant-tasting. It can be eaten plain by the teaspoonful, added to milkshakes, or sprinkled on desserts and confections. Most health food stores carry pollen from several different kinds of plants, such as Spanish gold, almond blossom, and mixed wildflowers. If you are gathering your own pollen, any plant which makes a good honey—such as sage, orange blossom, clover, tupelo, or fireweed—also yields an edible pollen. Pollen from poisonous plants such as yellow jasmine, foxglove and oleander should be avoided, as the toxins often concentrate in the pollen.

PUMPKIN SEEDS

The ripe seeds of the common pumpkin (*Cucurbita pepo*). These are an excellent food, rich in proteins, carbohydrates, unsaturated fatty acids, phosphorus, and B vitamins. They also contain substances that are beneficial to the genito-urinary passages and which encourage production of male sex hormones. The Gypsies of Eastern Europe eat the raw seeds regularly because of their nutritional value and because they are aware that they prevent disorders of the prostate, promote sexual vigor, and preserve potency well into a man's later years. They are one of the finest aphrodisiac materials because they serve more as a high-powered nutrient than as a drug. Raw, shelled pumpkin seeds are available at most health food stores for about $1.50 per pound. They should be kept under refrigeration to prevent them from going rancid. Rancid foods destroy vitamin E in the body and may even accelerate the aging process.

RHINO HORN

According to Chinese tradition, one of the world's most powerful aphrodisiacs is the powdered horn of a mature rhinoceros. A mere pinch of this material taken internally is said to make a man erect with lust and a woman abandoned to passion. It is also said that the horns are so potent that liquids drunk from cups carved of them will fill one with heat and desire. Analysis of the horns by chemists in the USA has revealed no substance which could serve as an aphrodisiac. Nevertheless, the rhino horn market continues to be a profitable business. A grown rhino horn weighs about four pounds and sells for $8,000 or more. That is about $2,000 a pound. Several years ago, thieves broke into the zoological museum in Jakarta, Indonesia, and sawed the horns from seven stuffed rhinoceros heads. They had no trouble selling these for a small fortune. Each year in London, two hundred rhino horns are auctioned for around a million dollars. Although the question about the efficacy of rhino horn to make one horny remains open and undecided, the ability of this product to stimulate friendship is now becoming a matter of history. Since the 1962 border war between China and India, relations between the two nations have been strained and there has been no official trade. However, India has permitted the underground exportation of rhino horns. Now, the Indian government is even supervising the sale of the horns to China because it believes that this product will lead to improved trade relations. It is hoped that the possible use of rhino horns as an aphrodisiac will not result in a mass slaughter and near extinction of the rhinoceros.

SARSAPARILLA

The roots of the tropical American vine *Smilax officianalis*. It is used by Indians of Mexico, Central and South America to overcome physical weakness and impotence. Since sarsaparilla is a well-known flavoring agent in the USA, this use was thought to be nonsense. Then, in 1939, it was found that this root is rich in sterones. Now it is used as a commercial source of testosterone, the male sex hormone. Testosterone can bring on secondary sex characteristics when they are slow to develop, enlarge an underdeveloped penis, overcome impotence when this is due to physical rather than psychological causes, and improve the health, muscle tone, energy, and sex drive of older men. Sarsaparilla also contains progesterone and cortin. The latter is an adrenal hormone which aids in resisting infection and nervous depression. 2 to 3 heaping tablespoons of dried sarsaparilla root is added to 1 pint of simmering water for 5 minutes. It will foam, so don't let it boil over. Strain the liquid and drink it slowly, holding each sip in the mouth for a minute before swallowing. Testosterone tends to be destroyed by digestive acids and is best absorbed through the buccal lining of the mouth. 1 or 2 cups of this tea is taken in the morning and again before retiring. This treatment is continued for 1 or 2 weeks, then discontinued. If necessary, the treatment may be resumed for the same duration after a break of 2 to 4 weeks. Uninterrupted use of testosterone can develop into dependence, in which case the body may weaken or even shut down its ability to produce the hormone. What we must aim to do with this natural medicine is to give the body just enough help to regain its strength that it can produce its own hormone once more.

SAW PALMETTO

The fresh or dried berries of a stemless palm (*Serenoa repens*) which grows is Florida and other parts of southeastern USA. At least ¼ ounce of the dried berries or as many fresh ones should be eaten daily to realize their benefits. They are a tonic for glandular tissues, build strength after illness, and increase sperm production when taken regularly. They have been used successfully to reverse atrophy of the testes and mammary glands and to improve catarrhal soreness of the genito-urinary passages. Prolonged use sometimes increases the size of underdeveloped female breasts. They are most effective in all of these respects when damiana is also taken. They do not act as an aphrodisiac after a single use, but must be taken regularly for a while to build sexual vigor.

SENSITIVE PLANT

The shrub *Mimosa pudica* which grows in Mexico, Central and South America. It is often sold as a house plant in the United States. If the leaves are touched or lightly stroked they will immediately close up. The Indians of the Amazon soak the leaves in the root juices and apply them to their breasts and the soles of their feet. This, they say, gives them increased sexual power which can last through many orgasms. Supposedly the active substances are absorbed through the skin. It has been found that the roots of this and other South American species of *Mimosa* contain several psychoactive tryptamines. None of these tryptamines, however, have any reputation as sex stimulants.

SERPOLET

A plant of the mint family, *Thymus serpyllum,* also known as mother of thyme or brotherwort. Its odor and taste are very spicy. An infusion of the dried herb is used against cramps and nervous conditions. It has a specific action on the sexual organs of both men and women. It has been used successfully to treat nervous disorders from disturbances in these parts. In cases where there is excessive nervous tension in the genital area, serpolet may have an aphrodisiac-like effect by reducing this tension sufficiently that the sex act may be consummated and enjoyed.

SOUTHERNWOOD

A shrubby, fragrant European wormwood (*Artemisia abrotanum*) with a bitter-tasting foliage. An infusion of this herb is used as a stimulant for the heart and brain and as an aphrodisiac. It is also used to bring on delayed or scanty menstruation. The taste of the tea is pungent and somewhat bitter. It is also used internally in herbal medicine to induce perspiration, strengthen the digestive organs, overcome emaciation, and to treat convulsions and hysteria. Externally, it is applied as a lotion to prevent the falling-out of hair and even to promote hair growth.

SPANISH FLY

The pulverized wing parts of a species of beetle, *Lytta vesicatoria* (also *Cantharis vesicatoria*). It contains an irritant to animal tissues. Plasters made from these beetle wings have been used medically to raise blisters. Spanish fly, or cantharides as it is sometimes called, is often given orally to farm animals to incite them to mating. The cantharides excreted in the urine irritate the urethral passages, causing inflammation in the genitals which gives the illusion of sexual arousal. Spanish fly has also been given to human beings for purposes of seduction. This is very dangerous. The amount required is miniscule and the difference between the effective dose and the harmful dose is quite narrow. Cantharides cause painful urination, fever, and sometimes bloody discharge. They can easily cause permanent damage to the kidneys and genitals and may even result in death. Furthermore, they are not always likely to give sensations or erotic arousal. Most often they produce a painful and unpleasant experience.

Cantharides are illegal except for use in animal husbandry. Some sex drug companies attempting to capitalize on the reputation of Spanish fly as a potent aphrodisiac advertise such products as Mexican Spanish Fly, Original Spanish Fly, Real "Spanish Fly" Vitamin Tablets (the vitamins are real), Spanish Fly Potions, containing what they call "spurious cantharides" (this sounds intriguing if you do not know that the word *spurious* means false, counterfeit, fictitious, illegitimate). Most frequently the substance is actually capsicum (cayenne pepper), but never true Spanish fly.

STRYCHNINE

The active alkaloid derived from the seed of the tree *Strychnos nux vomica*, which grows in China, Burma, India and Australia. Used properly, strychnine is an effective medicine for the temporary relief of neuralgia, dyspepsia and impotence. In the case of impotence, its results are due to its stimulation of circulation, muscle tone, and the spinal nerves which produce erection. There is a narrow margin between the effective and dangerous doses. 2 mg can serve as a sexual stimulant. Larger amounts can cause rapid heart and pulse rate, convulsions, and possible death. Individual tolerances may vary. Medical supervision is recommended when using this drug.

Crude extracts of *Strychnos* seed are sometimes combined with other materials in the preparation of prescription and patent medicines for the treatment of impotence. An example of this is Aphrodex, which contains *Strychnos*, testosterone and yohimbine (see *Yohimbine Hydrochloride* for detailed description).

Strychnine can have such a profound influence on the spinal ganglia which control the erectile tissue that a man may suffer from a powerful and painful erection that refuses to subside even after several orgasms. Strychnine may also cause a person to develop strong body heat and abundant perspiration. However potent the drug might make a man, excessive sweat may dampen if not drown romantic sentiments. The author does not recommend the unsupervised use of *Strychnos* or strychnine and suggests that yohimbine and burra gokeroo have similar erection-stimulating properties, without the above-mentioned dangers.

VANILLA PODS

The long, capsular, fragrant fruit of the tropical climbing orchid *Vanilla planifolia*. Vanilla is a well-known article of commerce for the flavoring extract that it yields. The small quantity consumed in ice creams and pastries is insufficient to produce any physiological changes, but larger amounts of the raw material or pure extract can have definite aphrodisiacal results. It is said that the notorious Madame DuBarry fed vanilla to her lovers to keep them primed for lechery. How vanilla serves to excite one sexually is not well established, but it probably acts as a urethral irritant in the same manner as Spanish fly, only much more mildly. Workers who gather and handle vanilla pods often develop skin irritations, especially on their hands. It may be of interest to experiment occasionally with vanilla as a sex drug, but continued use is not advised. Any substance which can cause skin irritations is likely to have damaging effects on the internal organs, such as the liver and kidneys. For a starting dose, no more than one or two pods should be consumed.

Many scholars of Ancient Greek culture are convinced that the legendary Hellenic aphrodisiac known as *Satyrion* was the root of another type of orchid called *orchishircina*. This root was crushed and combined with goat's milk. He who drank it was supposed to gain the sexual prowess of a satyr.

VIRGINIA SNAKE ROOT

The root of the vine *Aristolochia serpentaria*. It has an aromatic odor resembling valerian, but less pungent. In the form of an infusion or tincture, it has been used as a stimulant-tonic and to induce the flow of perspiration and urine. Combined with cinchona bark (the source of quinine), it has been used to treat certain infections and fevers. This combination has also been employed as a sedative for the genital nerves. In cases where nervous tension in the genital area prevents successful copulation, the combination of these two drugs, and sometimes the addition of serpolet (*Thymus serpyllum*), may make sexual intercourse possible. A tea can be made by boiling one heaping tablespoon each of Virginia snake root and cinchona bark in a pint of water for ten minutes and then pouring this brew over a heaping tablespoon of serpolet and allowing this to steep for five minutes before straining.

VITAMIN E

Any of over one hundred related compounds from the tocopherol group. These are oil-soluble compounds found in wheat germ, unrefined vegetable oils, nuts, seeds, and leafy vegetables. Alpha-tocopherol is the most active compound of the series, but the other compounds, as contained in preparations labeled "mixed tocopherols", are necessary for the proper function of this vitamin. In 1922 Evans demonstrated that deficiency of vitamin E produced sterility in rats.

As a result the substance was promoted as "the sex vitamin". To a great extent it has been overrated as such. However, the vitamin has several beneficial influences upon sexual health. It is found in greatest concentration in the anterior pituitary gland, where it positively influences the production of male sex hormones. It also protects these hormones and other vital substances in the body against oxidation. It improves heart response and thereby gives the user greater physical endurance. It also helps to break up accumulations of arterial cholesterol and to conserve oxygen in the blood. For these reasons, it may increase a person's sexual capacity, especially if he has previously been somewhat deficient in the vitamin. Extreme deficiency can lead to weakness of the muscle tissues, disorders of the reproductive system, irreversible degeneration of the testes, sterility, miscarriage, stillbirth, and spontaneous abortion. This vitamin has been used to relieve unpleasant menopause symptoms, including backache, excessive menstruation, hot flashes, high blood pressure, and muscular discomfort.

Vitamin E is apparently non-toxic. Doses of 400 to 1600 units daily can be taken to good advantage without side effects. Oil-soluble vitamins are best taken after a large meal containing fats or oils. Under these circumstances, there is sufficient bile flow to assimilate the vitamins. Capsules or pearls containing mixed tocopherols in oil form are recommended far above the synthetic and water-dispersible forms. Five times as much of the synthetic vitamin is required to achieve the same results as can be had from the natural product.

Persons suffering from extreme high blood pressure or heart damage from chronic rheumatic fever should not take large amounts of vitamin E without supervision of a qualified physician. In such cases, the standard procedure is to start with daily doses of 50 units and increase by 25 units every six weeks. Persons who are afflicted with overactive thyroid or who are taking insulin or digitalis should consult a physician before taking large doses of this vitamin.

WILD MINT

The aromatic leaves of the herbaceous plant *Mentha sativa*. In ancient Greece a strong tea made from the fresh or recently dried leaves of this plant was believed to arouse erotic desire in both males and females. So strong was this belief that on the advice of his tutor Aristotle, Alexander the Great forbade his troops the use of this tea during times of war. Like other wise men and generals of his time, he felt that wild mint tea heightened sexual desire and softened courage and the will to fight. A similar attitude was held about the excessive use of thyme and rosemary. Mint tea was made stronger and consumed in greater quantities than it is today. To prepare mint tea in the ancient way, bring the water to a boil, remove it from the heat for one minute, then pour one pint of water over two ounces of dried mint leaves and allow to soak for five minutes with a cover over the teapot. Never boil mint leaves or you will evaporate away the essential oils.

YAGE

Pronounced YAH-hay; a brew prepared from the bark of the South American jungle liana *Banisteriopsis cappi* or possibly one of several other species of *Banisteriopsis*. It contains the unusual psychoactive beta-carbolines harmine, harmaline, and *d*-tetrahydroharmine. It is used by natives of the Amazon and Orinoco regions for divination, and for its pleasurable and aphrodisiacal effects. Small amounts of the drug act as a psychic energizer and sex stimulant. Larger amounts can produce brilliant hallucinations, illusions of size changes of objects, and unusually keen night vision. Excessive amounts can produce nightmare visions and a psychotic state.

Many persons have noted an increase in ESP ability while under the drug. The alkaloid harmine was formerly called telepathine. In South America the Indians prepare yage—or *ayahuasca,* as it is sometimes called—by boiling the bark in water with various other plant material containing such active components as DMT (dimethyltryptamine) and tropane alkaloids (belladonna alkaloids like atropine and scopolamine). These tropanes tend to augment the effects of the harmful alkaloids. A typical cup of yage used by these natives contains about 400 mg of combined harmal alkaloids. The cup is drunk and the drinker soon vomits most of the materials. Actually one can obtain the same psychic effects with much less of the drug. The harmal alkaloids are absorbed very poorly through the stomach and intestines. Conducting experiments on himself, the author has found that 25 to 100 mg of harmine hydrochloride can be taken as a snuff to produce almost immediate results. Unfortunately the drug produces a terrible burning of the nostrils and throat, which leaves one for several days with all of the nose and throat symptoms of a cold. Finally it was found that the best way to use the pure alkaloid is to place the same amount of the substance under the tongue and between the gums and the lips where it is readily absorbed.

The harmal alkaloids are most effective if used in combination rather than singly. All of the harmal alkaloids act upon the central nervous system. One of them, 6-methoxytetrahydroharmine, is found in the pineal gland of humans and other animals. There is some belief that this chemical is somewhat more abundant in the pineal of highly advanced yogis and that its presence imparts power to the so-called third eye.

In laboratory experiments, rats which had been given 5 mg of harmine showed a marked increase in sexual activity. Similar results were observed when the animals were given other harmal alkaloids such as harmaline and harmalol. None of these facts are particularly surprising when it is realized that the Indians of South America have for many generations used yage as a sexual stimulant. These people also employ the brew in their coming-into-manhood ceremonies. Flagellation and various erotic activities also figure into these rituals.

Syrian rue is another plant which contains harmine, harmaline and harmalol. This plant, known botanically as *Peganum harmala,* is found throughout the Mediterranean area, and in parts of the Middle East, Central Asia and North Africa. It spreads rapidly once it gets started and then is difficult to get rid of. Somehow, large patches of it got started in parts of Texas and the American southwest. Although the plant is not illegal, local authorities have tried to remove it as a noxious weed, but with little success.

It is the roots and seeds which contain the alkaloids. But the root is almost never used. The seeds have much commercial value, however. Turkish red dye, the pigment used in Turkish and Persian carpets, is made from the seeds. In Egypt the oil extracted from the seeds is sold for both aphrodisiacal and hallucinogenic purposes under the name Zit-el-Harmel. The seeds have also had considerable use as a folk medicine and condiment.

Two other plants which contain harmal alkaloids are *Zygophyllum fabago,* which can be found in the western United States, and passionflower *(Passiflora incarnata),* which grows in temperate areas throughout the world.

YOHIMBE

The inner bark of the tropical West African tree *Corynanthe yohimbe.* A tea is brewed of 6 teaspoons of shaved bark in 1 pint of boiling water for 10 minutes, strained, and sipped slowly 1 or 2 hours before coitus. Addition of 500 mg vitamin C strengthens and hastens action. The tea is not very pleasant-tasting. Honey may be added. The material contains several indole-based alkaloids, of which yohimbine is the most prominent. It causes increased vasodilation and peripheral blood flow in combination with stimulation of the spinal ganglia which controls the corpus spongiosum (erectile tissue). This action produces erections in the male. Other pleasurable effects are warm spinal shivers, which are especially enjoyable during coitus and orgasm (bodies feel like they are melting into one another), psychic stimulations, mild perceptual changes without hallucination, and heightening of emotional and sexual feeling. Effects last about two hours.

Yohimbine is also a mild serotonin inhibitor. It has been found that when larger than normal amounts of serotonin are produced in the body, blood pressure, nervousness, depression, and exhaustion are increased. There is also likely to be a loss of interest in sex. There is a possibility that some forms of impotence are not psychologically based or due to any waning of one's glandular manhood, but may simply be the result of increased serotonin levels in the brain. Conversely, substances which inhibit serotonin are likely to have an apparent aphrodisiacal influence. This response, however, is in fact the natural sex chemistry of the body being liberated pharmaceutically from the blockage of the serotonin.

Normally there are no undesirable after-effects. Individuals with sensitive stomachs may experience some queasiness or mild nausea for a few minutes shortly after drinking the tea. It is best to sip it slowly. Yohimbe should not be used by persons suffering from blood pressure disorders, diabetes, hypoglycemia, or active ailments or injury of kidneys, liver or heart. It is a brief-acting monoamine oxidase inhibitor and should not be used by persons under the influence of alcohol, amphetamines (even diet pills), antihistamines, narcotics, or certain tranquilizers

(Librium is ok). Yohimbe may cause insomnia in some persons if taken too near retiring.

YOHIMBINE HYDROCHLORIDE

The hydrochloride salt of the main active alkaloid in yohimbe bark. It usually comes as a fluffy white powder with very little taste. 5 to 20 mg can be ingested, placed beneath the tongue or around the inner cheeks, or snorted, for approximately the same effects as yohimbe gives. The cautions mentioned under yohimbe are equally applicable. The inclination towards nausea is less likely if the material is snorted. Bentex Pharmaceutical Company, Houston, Texas, produces a pill called Afrodex, which has been useful in treating male impotence. Each capsule contains 5 mg yohimbine hydrochloride, 5 mg methyltestosterone, and 5 mg *nux vomica* extract. The standard dose is 1 capsule 3 times daily. For best results the capsule should be opened and the contents placed beneath the tongue where it can be absorbed. Methyltestosterone is one of the major male hormones. Continued use of this hormone may create dependence resulting in a shutdown of the body's ability to produce its own sex hormones. It is mainly intended for those who have passed male climacteric (change of life). Younger men suffering temporary impotence stemming from recent illness or psychological causes should not continue the use of this hormone more than two weeks. *Nux vomica* is the source of strychnine. This alkaloid can be effective in stimulating male erection when used in small doses (2 mg orally). In larger doses it is a very dangerous poison.

Formulary
of
Herbal Blends

FORMULARY OF HERBAL BLENDS

1. For firm erection (Chemical compound)

Yohimbine Hydrochloride	5 mg.
Methyltestosterone	5 mg.
Pemoline	25 mg.
Strychnine Sulfate	2 mg.

The ingredients are blended and put into a gelatin capsule. The capsule is opened and its contents placed under the tongue one hour before intercourse. Warning: persons suffering from disorders of the heart, liver or kidneys should not use this compound.

2. For firm erection (Herbal Compound)

Yohimbe Bark (shaved)	1 tbsp.
Dita Seed (crushed)	½ tsp.
Kola Nuts (broken)	1 tbsp.
Sarsaparilla Bark (shaved)	1 tbsp.

The ingredients are boiled for 10 minutes in one pint of water, care being taken to avoid frothing and boiling over. One or two cups of brew is sipped slowly one hour before intercourse.

3. For increased sexual energy

> Capsicum (powdered)
> Ginseng (powdered)
> Gotu Kola (powdered)
> Guarana (powdered)

Equal parts of the ingredients are thoroughly blended and put up in large (00) gelatin capsules. One or two capsules are taken with a cup of warm water one hour before intercourse.

4. For increased sexual energy (Luv-Mu-Tea)

Calamus (broken)	1 oz.
Muira Puama (shaved)	2 oz.
Ginseng (broken)	1 oz.
Vanilla Pods (chopped)	3 pods
Kola Nuts (broken)	2 oz.
Betel Nuts (broken)	½ oz.
Southernwood (shaved)	1 oz.
Yohimbe Bark (shaved)	1 oz.
Nutmeg (broken)	2 nuts
Cloves (whole)	½ oz.

The ingredients are combined homogeneously and stored in a sealed container under refrigeration. ½ oz. is boiled for 5–10 minutes in a 4-cup pyrex coffee maker. One or more cups are drunk one hour before intercourse. A second and possibly third pot may be prepared by adding fresh water to the remaining pulp and boiling for slightly longer periods.

5. Tonic tea for genital health and strength plus increased sperm production (Afro-Dee-Tee)

Cubeb Leaves	1 oz.
Damiana	2 oz.
Ginseng	1 oz.
Gotu Kola	2 oz.
Fleeceflower Root	1 oz.
Saw Palmetto Berries	2 oz.
Calamus	1 oz.
Sarsaparilla	1 oz.
Buchu Leaves	2 oz.
Serpolet	2 oz.
False Unicorn Root	1 oz.

All ingredients are purchased in powdered form. To blend, combine herbs in a 2-pound coffee can, cap it, and shake vigorously for 5 minutes. 1 or 2 teaspoons of this powder are placed in a cup and made into a slurry by moistening with hot water and stirring. More hot water is added to fill the cup. 1 to 3 cups of this tea may be taken daily over a period of 2 to 8 weeks for increasing sexual vigor, sperm production, and genital tone.

6. To prevent premature ejaculation

Lupuline (sifted from dried hops)
Dita Seeds (crushed or powdered)
Serpolet (powdered)
Cinchona Bark (powdered)
Virginia Snakeroot (powdered)
False Unicorn Root (powdered)

Equal parts of the ingredients are blended thoroughly. 1 level teaspoon of blend is slurried with hot water in a cup, which is then filled with hot water and drunk in large sips one hour before intercourse, or the same amount can be put up in 2 or 3 large gelatin capsules, which are swallowed with a cup of warm water 90 minutes to 2 hours before intercourse.

7. For sexual revitalization

Gotu Kola Leaves	1 oz.
Sarsaparilla (broken)	2 oz.
Licorice (broken)	2 oz.
Cotton Root (broken)	1 oz.
Ginseng (broken roots)	2 oz.
Cereus grandiflorus (fresh and crushed)	½ oz.

The first four ingredients are soaked in one quart of vodka for 10 days. Then the liquor is strained. The ginseng and fresh Cereus grandiflorus are put in the bottle with the liquor and stored for at least 10 days before using. 1 ounce (shot glass) is taken once or twice daily for one week or 30 minutes before intercourse to combat sexual lassitude and to revitalize libido after sexual exhaustion.

Mail Order
Suppliers

REASONABLY PRICED
MAIL ORDER
SUPPLIERS

When ordering from any of the following companies, please observe these suggestions:

1) Send first for their catalogue. Enclose 50 cents to cover postage.

2) Inquire about products not listed before attempting to order them. State both common and Latin names of plants, seeds or herbs to avoid error.

3) Do not use such terms as sex drug, aphrodisiac, stimulant, or psychedelic when corresponding with these companies. Do not inquire about dosages, methods of use or pharmacological effects of any materials which they sell. FDA rulings forbid vendors of herbs to prescribe herbs for any pharmacological purposes or to make any claims as to their usage or effects.

Most of the herbal materials described in this book are available from the following addresses:

The Magic Garden Herb Co., P.O. Box 332, Fairfax, CA 94930.

Harvest Health, Inc., 1944 Eastern Avenue S.E., Grand Rapids, MI 49507.

East Earth Herb Co., Rt. 3, Box 181, Reedsport, OR 97467.

A mixture of 90 to 95 percent pure yohimbine hydrochloride balanced with corynanthine and other natural yohimbe alkaloids is available in a product called Yocaine. For a 100-mg sample and information, send $3 to Paracelsus, Inc., P.O. Box 93, Barrington, NJ 08007.

Pangamic acid tablets are available at some health food stores in states which do not forbid its sale. It is sometimes sold under the counter to preferred customers in California health food stores. It can be ordered from Natural Nutritional, P.O. Box 448, Passaic, NJ 07055.

Live gotu kola plants are available from:

Thomas A. David, Independent Scientific Research, 19886 Geer Avenue, Hilmar, CA 95324.

Live *Cereus grandiflorus* cuttings are available from:

A. Hugh Dial, 7587 Deer Trail, Yucca Valley, Calif.

New Mexico Cactus Research, P.O. Box 787, Belen, New Mexico.

Seeds for many of the plants mentioned in this book are available from:

Redwood City Seed Co., P.O. Box 361, Redwood City, CA 94061.

Chemicals described in this book are available from many companies throughout the United States. Rather than attempt to list them all, we will recommend that the reader refer to the annual listing entitled *Chemical Sources USA*. It can be found on the reference shelf at most large libraries, especially at universities and colleges; or it may be purchased from the publishers, *Directories Publishing Company, Inc.*, Flemington, New Jersey. One may look up any chemical in this catalogue and find numerous suppliers listed for it.

Two typical mail order sex drug companies which advertise through the sexually oriented underground tabloids are Cru-tri-cir Corp., P.O. Box 507, Reseda, CA 91335 and Herbal Holding Co., P.O. Box 5854, Sherman Oaks, CA 91413, and a typical legitimate mail order herb dealer is Magic Garden Herb Co., P.O. Box 332, Fairfax, CA 94930. In most cases the capsules mentioned contain about 8 grains of materials. 50 capsules contain about 1 oz. of materials. 100 capsules equals about 2 oz. Yohimbine tabs as sold by Herbal Holding Co. weigh 5 grains each. 100 of these tabs equal about 1⅛ oz. The damiana sold by Herbal Holding Co. is blended with saw palmetto berries. These berries sell for $4.50 per lb. at Magic Garden Co., and are about the same price from most regular herb dealers.

The names and formulas for the products: *Super Vita-Shake, Afro-Dee-Tee* and *Luv-Mu-Tea* are original with the author and may not be used commercially without written permission from him.

Printed in the USA
CPSIA information can be obtained
at www.ICGtesting.com
JSHW012056140824
68134JS00035B/3474